HOW TO LOSE WEIGHT WITH THE GASTRIC BALLOON PROGRAM

MY SECRETS AND TIPS TO A SUCCESSFUL JOURNEY!

Sabine Fontaine

supportgballoon@outlook.com

https://www.facebook.com/pages/Losing-Weight-with-the-Gastric-Balloon-Program/673321786040499

Also by Sabine Fontaine:

My Successful Gastric Balloon Diet
- 4 Steps to Lose Weight and Keep it Off!

How to Lose Weight at Christmas
with the Gastric Balloon

Published by Sabine Fontaine

Copyright © 2013 Sabine Fontaine

All rights reserved worldwide

ISBN:9781496051394

No part of this publication may be stored in a retrieval system, transmitted, or reproduced in any way, including, but not limited to, digital copying without the prior agreement and written permission of the author.

Disclaimer

The author and publisher, Sabine Fontaine, has made every effort to produce a high-quality, informative, and helpful book. However, she makes no representation or warranties of any kind with regard to the completeness or accuracy of the content of the book. She accepts no liabilities of any kind for any losses or damages caused or alleged to be caused, directly or indirectly, from using the information contained in this book.

It is the first book of its kind. There has been no book dedicated to providing a full experience on how life is with the gastric balloon.

This book is not intended to be a substitute for nutritional advice and/or sessions you are encouraged to attend.

Although the author has qualified in nutrition, her aim is to help, guide and give ideas on what has worked for her.

Foreword

Obesity is on the increase, and yet, diets as well as invasive and non-invasive procedures aiming at losing weight flourish. This is a global phenomenon and has become endemic.

My name is Nadey Hakim, I am a Consultant Surgeon and professor of Surgery, the Surgical Director of the Transplant Unit at Imperial College Healthcare NHS Trust London. I have a particular interest in kidney and pancreas transplantation and in Bariatric surgery. I have written and published papers and textbooks, including "Bariatric Surgery" from Imperial College Press, a book in which there is a dedicated chapter on the BioEnterics Intragastric Balloon.

Patients consult me first to go through the different options offered to them. They rarely know what solution they want to opt for.

The adjustable gastric band also called Lapband, the Gastric sleeve and Gastric Bypass are routine procedures we have all read about on blogs, websites or books. Although most of us have also heard about the gastric balloon, we haven't read about it, or at least, there has been no dedicated book written on the subject so far, as the procedure is less known than others. However I have already performed over 2500 of these procedures. Therefore, I believe this book will be well received amongst patients.

This volume is the first of its kind and describes the journey from the moment you have decided to have a gastric balloon fitted until the last day it is removed. It's a step by step guide and it takes you through all the decisions you will have to make and much more. It explains the possible symptoms you might experience while having the gastric balloon.

In my practice, the rate of success ranges from 70 to 85%; this guide is useful and intuitive. There is another book dedicated to recipes, also the first of its kind so far which will complement this book.

My patients have been waiting for a gastric balloon guide that would adequately answer all the questions they have. In truth, we all know that the least understood procedure is prone to generate more questions.

Before patients have the gastric balloon fitted, I have a conversation with them, which encompasses the various concerns and questions they might have.

Sabine lost approximately 4 stone with the gastric balloon; she, too, had a lot of questions for me before she started her journey, right after I have inserted the balloon, and over the 26 weeks she had it in situ.

The average weight loss of my patients varies according to their lifestyle and the way they manage to treat the root cause of the issues that have overtaken their lives enough to be willing to undergo this non-invasive solution.

The journey is more than simply a medical device; it is a program helping weight loss thanks to the gastric balloon, a balanced diet, physical exercise and the understanding and healing, through your preferred holistic method, of the underlying root cause of excessive weight.

I would invite you to read this successful journey put together so brilliantly by Sabine, and why not, make an informed decision to have the gastric balloon fitted yourself.

Good luck.

NH

Acknowledgments

This book was conceived after many friends and acquaintances encouraged me to share my successful experience with others, and I would like to thank them.

My deepest thanks go to a dear friend of mine, who also happens to be the proofreader of my two first books on the gastric balloon, Tracy Bullock. Tracy is simply fabulous. The quality of her work is remarkable, and her friendship has been instrumental in the writing of this series of books on the gastric balloon.

My deepest thanks go to another dear friend of mine, Rony Sidon, who is the amazing artist who designed the internal characters. Rony was patient enough to adapt his wonderful style to my requirements. I am thrilled with the results as it is both artistic—while self-explanatory with regard to the power of the mind—and it highlights the gastric balloon as a tool connecting the mind to foods.

My deepest thanks go to another dear friend of mine, Samantha Long. Her patience has been exemplary and, being an excellent friend, she encouraged me during that journey and congratulated me on my progress. Working with Samantha was great as she was there every step of the way.

My deepest thanks go to Luanne, who formatted my book in a timely manner, and to Tommy, who designed the cover in a split of a second.

My deepest thanks go to many friends who have contributed to this book, in one way or another, by supporting my journey, by encouraging me, and by sharing tips with me, the examples are endless.

I would like to start by offering my heartfelt thanks to Giuliano Zorzan, as well as Luca Balicco and Delia MK for their so appreciated encouragements and constant great advice on this project; Mairead Adams, David Caharel, David

Jaureguiberry, Sandrine Marchandon, and Philippe Lacroix for being there when I needed them, to name but a few.

Heartfelt thanks go to Elisa Rampinini, Stephanie Taranne, Delphine Chauveau, and Claire Lasfargues for their close friendship and support.

My deepest thanks go to Professor Nadey Hakim and his outstanding team who have made my successful journey possible; I feel lucky to have been in such good hands. Professor Hakim has also honoured me with the foreword of this book and I am humbled by his encouragements.

Last, but not least, my deepest thanks go to my parents who have supported me throughout, way and beyond this exciting journey, and have encouraged me at all times.

Table of Contents

Introduction — 1

Chapter One — 5
Methods I Have Tried Throughout the Years and Their Results — 5

Chapter Two — 7
What Is the Gastric Balloon? — 7

Chapter Three — 8
What Is the Difference with a Gastric Band? — 8

Chapter Four — 9
Why Choose the Gastric Balloon Over Another Method? — 9
Why am I convinced it is uniquely working? — 10
A word on vitamins and minerals — 11

Chapter Five — 13
Is the Intra-Gastric Balloon For You? — 13

Chapter Six — 15
Where To Go and For What Price? — 15
What are the costs involved? — 15
Location, location: how to choose — 17

Chapter Seven — 21
What Is the Gastric Balloon Program? — 21
Gastric balloon and support group — 21
Gastric balloon and individual therapy — 21
Gastric balloon and nutritionist sessions — 22

Chapter Eight — 24
Get Ready for the Gastric Balloon — 24
How to prepare best a month pre-procedure — 24
How to prepare best a week pre-procedure — 25
What to do the day prior to the procedure — 27
D-Day, what does the procedure entail? — 28

Chapter Nine — 31
The First Day's Post Procedure — 31
What are the possible symptoms? — 31
How to deal with them — 31

Chapter Ten — 33
What Are the Symptoms Within the First Three Months? — 33
- *What are the possible symptoms/side effects?* — 33
- *How to deal with them* — 33

Chapter Eleven — 37
The Last Remaining Months with the Gastric Balloon — 37
- *Possible symptoms/side effects and how to overcome them* — 37

Chapter Twelve — 39
Your Last Day with the Gastric Balloon — 39

Chapter Thirteen — 40
Keep Up Your Great Efforts and Make It a Lifelong Journey! — 40
- *Make your healthy life a long-lasting routine* — 40
- *Attend an additional therapy session if under pressure* — 41

Chapter Fourteen — 42
What Is the Plateau? — 42
- *Do we all hit the plateau?* — 42
- *Why do we hit the plateau with the gastric balloon program?* — 43
- *How to counteract the plateau* — 45

Chapter Fifteen — 50
Some Physical Exercise — 50
- *A word on sport* — 50

Chapter Sixteen — 54
Travelling Tips — 54
- *Tips if you travel* — 54
- *Tips for short hauls* — 55
- *Tips for long hauls* — 58

Conclusion — 59

About the Author — 61

Introduction

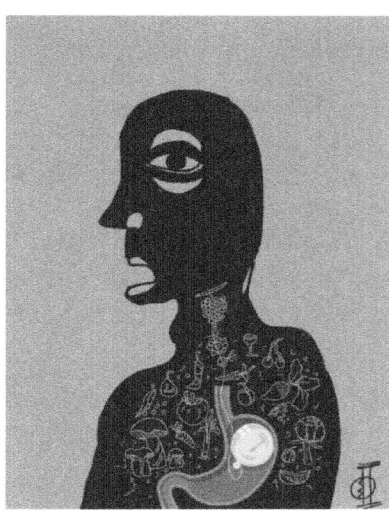

"Diet? Not when a gastric balloon will get weight off faster"[...] titled Tom Anderson in his article dated Sunday, 1 January 2006 in The Independent, London, UK.

This book is intended for those who are going to live with the gastric balloon for six months or want to assess if this is the right program for them.

My journey with the gastric balloon started in February 2008 in the UK.

At the time, I looked for any material that would help me understand what I would go through; it has been quite a challenge to find a handbook or any FAQs to live that period to the fullest.

I wanted to fully assess:

- If the balloon had a fair chance of success

- How much weight I was likely to lose
- How much I had to save to pay for it
- How much change in my life could be expected
- How to sustain the weight loss

Many websites mention uncomfortable physical symptoms but not how to deal with them. Listing them was reassuring in the sense that it drew a map of my expectations, but reading about solutions that would stop the physical symptoms would have been a great help.

- What were all the physically uncomfortable symptoms that websites were listing
- More importantly, how to deal with them without suffering from them
- Was there a list of food to avoid or a list of food to add
- Was there a list of liquids to avoid or add
- Was there any exercise to avoid doing
- When to eat—when not to eat
- When to drink—when not to drink

My questions were endless.

With all this in mind, I decided to compile all my notes based on my symptoms and solutions I found after a few trials, based on the answers from the surgical team, and based on information I could gather and experiment with.

I have also consulted many forums and have collated the questions to provide as broad a range of information and solutions to concerns shared by all who were living the same situation.

You might not experience all the symptoms described here. In fact, you might not experience them at their highest level, but it is my belief that commenting on them all or commenting on all the symptoms I have experienced at some stage, can only benefit you.

It is relatively easy for me to share this journey with you because your own experience is always easier to describe.

I know what you are going through and what you will go through, I understand your concerns, your questions, and your dreams. I have been there, I have done it, I have succeeded, but I feel that some guidance could have optimised my journey.

The gastric balloon is going to be part of your life for six months. In a lifetime, this is considered a very short period of time; however, you must have thought about it, talked about it and very soon, will live with it. After you have lived with it, you will probably want to stabilise the new you and the way you look and feel.

So what is considered a very short period of time within a lifetime suddenly becomes quite an important part of your life, wouldn't you agree?

So how about if you were considering the gastric balloon, not only as a tool to help you lose weight, but also as a friend or a friendly visitor who resides with you and whose aim is to help you live better?

Let's be really honest here: your new friend is also quite demanding and a fussy eater, but it's for your own good, I promise!

I have experienced this new life, this new lifestyle, and have come up with plenty of ideas to cohabit better with that new friend, adapt myself to it and be grateful for the new lifestyle it offered me. I also qualified post gastric balloon as a nutritionist—as mentioned earlier—as I wanted to know exactly what to eat and why.

I also studied the digestive system as well as the endocrine system in order to counteract better the symptoms I was experiencing, as I knew my digestion would be affected and my body would have to work harder now that there would be co-habitation with the balloon visitor.

Whether or not you are already adamant that you are going to embark on the balloon cruise, I would suggest that you read this book once first and then chapter by chapter as you go along.

By reading it once first, it will help you make informative decisions, have an overview of what the whole journey is going to look like, prepare yourself mentally—especially if you come across some topics that are new to you—and be ready to kick start your new life.

I would like to share my experience with you, and I can assure you that the journey with the gastric balloon and its program is really a second chance.

Chapter One

Methods I Have Tried Throughout the Years and Their Results

Over the years, through boredom and loneliness, I had gained 20 kilos that I was desperate to lose. In 2000, I also suffered from hormonal problems, which led to surgery, and a combination of lack of exercise and medication resulted in my gaining more weight. I was a wreck, trying to get back on my feet.

After a while, I had no control over what my body was absorbing, and I started to develop a real guilt around food.

I was consuming large quantities of food randomly and was starving myself at other times; I clearly had no idea how to get back to a healthy diet, a healthy me.

I started a chain of diets that worked for some time until I gave up and went back to my bad habits, regaining all the weight I had lost, even more sometimes. I'm pretty sure you're familiar with the protein diet, the Mediterranean diet, and the cabbage soup diet, to name but a few.

I do not intend to criticise any weight loss method; I did lose some weight with most of them, but it was far too easy for me to stop restricting myself and resume my pattern. And by resuming my eating patterns, the weight loss faded away within weeks, even days sometimes.

All in all, it was a vicious circle from which I could not see the end. I started to envision my life as a succession of diets and no promise of leading a healthy life.

In one magazine out of two, I could see miraculous ways of losing weight, magical pills promising to have the weight fall off me, ways to lose weight in fourteen days, sometimes in six days! All of them were very tempting, if you skip the bowel turmoil that is, but then what?

I finally came back to my senses and decided to lose weight steadily while ensuring it would be a long lasting method.

All I wanted was to go back to my original weight, or at least regaining a healthy BMI comprised between 18 and 25. I was aiming at a BMI of 24 to 25.

You probably know how to calculate your body max index by dividing your weight in kg by your height in square meters.

BMI = Weight (kg) / Height (m)^2.

You should aim at an ideal BMI being comprised between 18 and 25.

- Below 18 is considered underweight
- Between 25 to 30 is overweight
- Obese is from 30 to 35
- Severely obese is from 35 to 40 and finally
- Morbidly obese is a BMI greater than 40

By then, I had reached a BMI of 30.

Chapter Two

What Is the Gastric Balloon?

The gastric balloon—also called laparoscopic gastric balloon, intra gastric balloon, and stomach balloon—is a small soft and expandable balloon with a self-sealing valve; a thin tube or catheter is attached to it.

As far as I was aware, at the time of print, there were two kinds of gastric balloons: the air filled one and a liquid filled one.

I cannot recommend one device over the other; the decision is yours, although this will probably be recommended by your surgeon.

The usual timeline you are looking at is a six-month period, after which you get the gastric balloon removed.

More recently, I have read that there was an option to have the balloon left in the stomach for a twelve-month period. I personally got a silicon liquid filled intra gastric balloon for a six-month period.

The majority of clinics/hospitals that offer this program have diagrams on their website to illustrate what the gastric balloon looks like.

Chapter Three

What Is the Difference with a Gastric Band?

If you have opted for the gastric band, it is still at the stomach level that this is implemented, but as opposed to being inside the stomach, it is a small inflatable ring that is placed at the top of the stomach so that only small amounts of food will be able to pass through. You will not feel really hungry, similarly to the gastric balloon; the gastric band is adjustable and reversible. It is different from a bypass in that there are no staples.

The same concept applies here: you will have to take three lighter meals as well as two snacks. You will not have restrictions in terms of food, but I would urge you to follow the same diet as it has proven to be effective and work long term.

Both the gastric balloon and the gastric band have been developed to counteract weight problems or what is more commonly referred to as *obesity*.

Again, most of the websites related to gastric bands display images of the inflatable ring.

Chapter Four

Why Choose the Gastric Balloon Over Another Method?

The reason no diet was working for me was because I was not changing my eating habits, nor was I looking into the root cause of the real issue. I needed help and I needed focus. I needed a method that would lead me into changing my eating behaviours and removing the root cause of my being overweight in the first place.

I wanted a long-term, a long-life solution, not a quick fix.

As I pointed out previously, I had a BMI of 30. If you have opted for that system, you are likely to have a body mass index comprised between, say 27- 30, 30 plus, but below 40.

This is quite a wide range and, of course, this only reflects a bracket as this varies from skeleton to skeleton. In any case, you should aim to lose around fifteen per cent of your body weight within six months with the intra gastric balloon.

I studied various methods by looking on the internet, buying a plethora of books, and discussing it with close friends, family members, and colleagues.

After a long research, I finally decided to investigate the gastric balloon. What appealed to me was:

- It is a six months' process. This was great for me; after all, I knew that weight would not magically disappear within a week. Six months is a realistic enough period of time to adopt new, healthy eating habits.

- I knew that the balloon would reject fat, fizzy drinks, chocolate, ice cream, biscuits, etc. and I needed this to prevent cravings from happening. Again, six months to get rid of cravings is a reasonable period of time. This was a great motivator for me.
- I knew no general anaesthetic was required, and that was a major plus for me. Being sedated only was a relief.
- I knew it would be noninvasive—so no incision whatsoever.
- Visually, I knew I would start losing weight rather quickly, so a great boost and motivation for me.
- I am conscious of my body image and wanted to avoid saggy skin after weight loss. By losing weight gradually, I knew I would be less subject to having saggy skin.
- I knew that I would fill up rapidly, so I wouldn't be thinking about food all the time, nor would I be tempted to eat randomly to avoid boredom or loneliness. Satiety would be almost immediate.

I have been asked what the difference is between the gastric balloon and an appetite suppressant. Appetite suppressants give a satiety feeling without rejecting fatty foods and fizzy drinks. The gastric balloon does. So, to me, it's a winner all along!

Why am I convinced it is uniquely working?

Let me start by sharing with you the relationship between a hormone called ghrelin and the hypothalamus.

In the magazine, *New Scientist*, published 5 September 2009 and titled "Gone Appétit," there is a fascinating article on pages 30 to 33 entitled "Full without Food."

The science writer Claire Ainsworth writes: [...Our digestive system produces both hormones that make you hungry, or sated. Ghrelin, produced by the lower part of the stomach, is a powerful promoter of hunger, while the small intestine releases a number of hormones when it senses the presence of food...]. She adds: [...shrinking the stomach seems to reduce ghrelin production, which would curtain hunger signals.].

The science writer is referring to the bypass in her article, but it is my belief that the gastric balloon has the same sub effect. After all, the capacity of food that the stomach can hold is reduced by sharing its space with the device; so in essence, to me it is similar in concept.

Besides, if it wasn't the case, that would mean that after the effects felt and experienced right after the procedure and lasting up to a maximum of seven days—with the nausea, vomiting, inability to eat, fluid intake increase—you wouldn't be able to eat as much due to the capacity reduction of the stomach, BUT you would still feel hungry, right?

Well, the fact is, we don't feel hungry at all and sometimes we have to be reminded to eat!

So, for me, this theory fits and happens to be working pretty well.

A word on vitamins and minerals

Why are vitamins and minerals important?

At first, when you have the balloon fitted, you will experience some tiredness, due in part to the fact that you will not be eating as much, if you were eating much before, and in any case, because you will inevitably be changing your dietary habits.

It is very important to choose a multivitamin that is going to not only keep your energy at a good level, but also participate in your new healthy eating.

In that respect, I would recommend a vitamin that contains:

Chromium and vitamin D—in order to assimilate sugar better. In other words, they regulate insulin.

Potassium—in order to avoid water retention

Iodine—in order to regulate the thyroid

Vitamin C—in order to burn more fat

Vitamin Bs (2/3/5/6)—to promote good thyroid functions

Chapter Five

Is the Intra-Gastric Balloon For You?

Each individual is unique; therefore, you might have been recommended the gastric balloon as the ideal solution:

- To lose weight from weight gained over the past few years
- To get some weight loss after other diet attempts have failed
- If you need to follow a strict program and have struggled in the past to follow a diet up to completion
- If you require a surgical procedure such as a bypass for instance, you might have been requested to first lose weight with the gastric balloon in order to alleviate risks/complications sometimes associated with a more invasive procedure
- If you are not eligible for surgical procedures

We are talking eligibility here, not motivation factors. You could be willing to lose weight because:

- Your doctor has recommended a course of action to dissipate some diseases
- You want to resume having an exercise routine and the extra weight makes it difficult
- You want to become pregnant and being above the "healthy" BMI range can be challenging in that respect
- You are getting married in the coming months

- Your child is getting married in the coming months
- You want to feel good about yourself again
- This is your personal project for the current year

Whatever the reason behind your choice, you will need that motivation to live this experience as nicely as possible. It really helps to think about your goal when you feel depleted at times.

In some cases, however, the gastric balloon will be refused if:

- You have an addiction to alcohol or drugs
- You are under 18 years of age
- You are being currently prescribed antibiotics, or aspirin, or corticoids, or anti-coagulants
- You are pregnant or considering getting pregnant while on the gastric balloon
- You have had previous gastrointestinal surgery, anomalies at the oesophagus
- You have suffered from any heart problems within the previous six months
- You suffer from thyroid, bowel, depression, schizophrenia, diabetes diseases

I believe that to be quite an exhaustive list of the main ailments I had to clear with my physician during our first meeting.

As a standard precaution, the nurse who prepped me right before surgery cleared the very same ailments with me.

Chapter Six

Where To Go and For What Price?

What are the costs involved?

This is a recurrent question I have seen on many forums. From what I could read on forums and after discussing it with a few people or being asked to recommend a location, I have come to realise that the decision to have the procedure done either in the UK or in Australia, for instance, as opposed to another country, is often financially motivated.

This is why I am discussing both topics in the same chapter, as location and price are often interrelated.

Wherever you have the procedure done, please be aware that the initial costs for the placement and removal of the device will include:

- The intra gastric balloon fees (the cost depends on the sort of balloon you choose—as mentioned in chapter three)
- The pre and post procedures nursing fees
- The operation room fees
- The anaesthetic fees
- The surgeon's fees
- The recovery room (usually private or semi-private)

Again, fees include both procedures, that is, the placement and removal of the device.

Many clinics offer easy instalment payments. When that is the case, it is often interest free and they offer different packages to choose from.

You need to enquire what is comprised in those fees, as the whole package may well be included: the placement and removal of the device fees plus the aftercare with nutritional advice, support group, and individual monthly psychological or therapy sessions.

I need to mention that most of the clinics do not divulge their detailed price online, but you can find that information out by calling them or filling in their free quotation directly on their website.

<u>In the UK</u>, an average would be £5,000 (although I have seen prices specifying "from" £3,950). I have also seen prices rising up to £6,500, and they included a hospital stay.

<u>In Australia</u>, I have researched pricing and have read on many occasions that the average costs would be $6,000 AUD.

<u>In Canada</u>, I have seen prices averaging $8500 CAD.

<u>In India</u>, costs would be in the region of $4900 USD as far as my researches indicate.

<u>In Eastern Europe</u>, and more specifically in Prague, lots of gastric balloon users have reportedly paid $4000 USD.

<u>In the USA</u>, after researching that information, I believe that the gastric balloon procedure is not widely performed there unfortunately.

What we can safely assume overall, after researching, is that costs seem lower in Latin America and Eastern Europe.

Location, location: how to choose

We have just talked about the usual fees the procedure itself would entail.

With the costs involved, I know that many have chosen or are considering having the procedure done abroad. Some countries such as Mexico, Brazil, Colombia, Germany, Belgium, Poland, and the Czech Republic, to name but a few, offer lower costs.

Aside from the regular fees listed above, you should take into account other expenses, such as:

- The cost of the flights
- A night's stay (although some clinics do include that cost in their overall quotation)
- You also need to consider the six months' period in terms of:
- How about the support group you are supposed to attend?
- How about the nutritionist who is usually recommended through the clinic and needs to follow your progress closely?
- How about, and this is critical, trust me, the therapy sessions you normally are being advised to undertake?

I was recommended by a colleague in charge of the medical device department, a well-known surgeon and professor on Harley Street, London UK: Professor Nadey Hakim.

I admit I was lucky. Professor Hakim assessed if it was indeed the best solution for me and if I was fitting the rules/criteria to adhere to the program—as mentioned in chapter five.

My surgeon was focusing on the physical aspect of the method, of course, and he put my mind at ease by answering my immediate questions.

This is a very important step if you do decide to undergo this program: you need to be confident that the surgeon who will implant the gastric balloon in your stomach has the right credentials and that he/she takes the time to talk the method through with you.

I requested to have an overview of the day in question and was reassured by the quality of the anaesthetic and nursing teams. I researched both the surgeon and his clinic—both of which have an outstanding reputation. This data gave me the confidence and reassurance that I was making the right choice.

So, my choice was to stay in the UK. I will confess that I did not have to pay for everything as I previously mentioned; I was referred by a colleague who was in charge of one of the devices. I might have had to make another decision if I had to pay the original price.

Of course, I cannot recommend a clinic over another one or a country over another one. It's everybody's individual choice, based on your budget and location preferences.

However, I thought I would simply mention that I have read a lot of posts in forums on the internet of people who were lamenting the fact that they had chosen a clinic overseas and were feeling isolated during the program.

Having said that, if you prefer to go ahead with the placement and removal of the device in another country, different from the country you reside in, I highly recommend that you still join a local or online support group. You also need to consult a nutritionist and, finally, facilitate the whole journey with the great help and guidance of a therapist.

Personally, I'm an advocate of a holistic therapy to complement the program. To me, this is critical to not only accelerate the weight loss, but also to guarantee a better success rate.

There are a number of alternative therapies that can be considered:

- CBT or Cognitive Behavioural Therapy: you get to understand your current behaviour towards food and adjust it accordingly to enhance your life

- Neuro-Linguistic Programming: usually combined with EFT and TFT (using tapping techniques), it's an overall therapy designed to change your self- limiting beliefs to a positive mind in order to achieve success in the issue you are facing

- Hypnotherapy: the practitioner finds the root cause of your current relationship with food before making positive suggestions to your subconscious

There are many more therapies to choose from.

Sometimes practitioners combine several methods as they all work towards the same goal: find the best possible approach that will effectively help you.

I've been asked why an alternative method was not sufficient, why the need of the gastric balloon?

I chose the gastric balloon simply because one needs to start somewhere, and it is my experience that most of the time, we want to aim at a device, at a pill, at a product, at a diet, before accepting to go for sessions.

We have a tendency to act on urgent issues in a logical manner: we need to lose weight. Fine, we know we need to eat smaller portions, eat less fat, eat less sugar, include more fruits and vegetables in our diet, and exercise more. We all know that and, yet, we look for the next-best option available in the market, the next most promising weight loss system. We tackle the weight loss for a while ... and then we're back to square one.

Logically speaking, when you talk about weight loss to your family, your friends, and your colleagues, do you actually discuss what the best alternative therapy to counteract weight loss is? Probably not.

This is why, to me, a device such as the gastric balloon is a great start to kick off the process. But, I need to stress that it is only the combination of the device, along with working with a support group, a dietician or a nutritionist, and a more medical or alternative therapy that will guarantee a long term success of the program.

Chapter Seven

What Is the Gastric Balloon Program?

Gastric balloon and support group

A support group is usually offered in the package. To be honest with you, mine was located too far away from where I live and I couldn't attend any sessions.

I felt so isolated that I decided to confide in friends, look at forums to ensure I was experiencing the same symptoms, and finally decided to study more about the digestive system altogether.

The point is, a support group is going to make you feel surrounded and liberating, as you will be able to share your experience and feel motivated by the sight of others in the same situation. It gives a great boost. In the absence of a local support group, I found comfort in another support network that targeted women with fuller figures.

Even though this group did not include any sit-in sessions as such, it was still beneficial at the time to be surrounded by like-minded individuals who also had weight issues.

Gastric balloon and individual therapy

The individual therapy is critical. I was on a budget and couldn't afford too many sessions, and I thought that the balloon on its own would do the job. However, a device is only what it is: a device.

It is a fantastic help, but long term is exactly like any other diet if you do not ally it with the rest of the method.

My weight loss lasted for over a year, then a great deal of stress took the best out of me and I started, despite my healthy routine during the balloon and my nutritional qualifications, to gain a bit of weight again.

By consulting my hypnotherapist, I'm happy to report though that I'm steadily losing weight and maintaining it.

Gastric balloon and nutritionist sessions

The nutritionist is a great guidance. Mine was specialised with the gastric balloon users so she knew in what emotional state I would be, the challenges I would face, and the inevitable adjustments I would need to make in my life.

What I discovered shocked me. In the first session, we discussed my eating habits and she simply looked at me and said, "The real problem here is dual. You are eating unhealthily, but above all, you are not eating enough." I nearly fell off the chair, because I was feeling guilty eating certain foods and, at times, I was not eating anything else outside those foods. This, in turn, led to a lack in vitamins and essential nutrients.

We all instinctively know what we should be eating and what we should avoid. But it is still quite surprising when we get to do a full "check-up" of our food consumption. And by this, I mean ALL our food and drink consumption on a daily basis over a week and over a month.

To sum up what we have just discussed, the gastric balloon program is MORE THAN A DEVICE. IT IS A COMPLETE WEIGHT AND BEHAVIOURAL CHANGING MANAGEMENT PROGRAM.

It is only by integrating all the ingredients that you will achieve the best recipe. Otherwise, the recipe can still taste good, but it will not look perfect or vice versa.

If you focus on yourself and on your body for a period of six months, <u>YOU WILL SUCCEED</u>.

This is the only program that has worked for me, despite all my prior attempts. And it would have worked in one go if I had followed it to the letter. I have learned my lesson and now I am food addiction free for life, and I love it!

Chapter Eight

Get Ready for the Gastric Balloon

How to prepare best a month pre-procedure

A month before you have the gastric balloon placed in your stomach, I would encourage you to check if you have the following symptoms:

- Do you feel bloated?
- Do you have abdominal pain?
- Do you suffer from haemorrhoids?
- Do you have episodes of diarrhoea alternated with constipation?
- Do you find yourself tired/lethargic?
- Do you feel nauseous?
- Do you have unusual episodes of flatulence?
- Do you have mood swings?

If you can answer yes to most of those symptoms, you might be suffering from a blocked and unhealthy colon. After alerting my GP about all of the symptoms I have just listed, I had an ultrasound, which revealed nothing, but then I was referred to have a colonoscopy, and that solved all of the symptoms described above.

The reason I am mentioning this to you at this stage is that when you live with the gastric balloon, chances are that you are going to feel bloated to begin with. If you are already bloated due to your colon being blocked, and suffer from other uncomfortable symptoms, you could complicate your life unnecessarily.

Also, remember that you need to ensure in the next six months that your digestion/digestive track is under control and is working to the best of its ability.

Besides, the cleansing process needs to be accompanied by the intake of certain foods and fluids, including citrus that can be too acidic when you are on the gastric balloon. As a consequence, it's a good idea to cleanse your colon prior to living with the gastric balloon and consequently maximise the weight loss through a healthy digestive and colon system.

This is by no means something I'm saying that you need to do, only that it could be wise to consider it should you experience the symptoms above.

There are different ways to cleanse your colon:

- Hydrotherapy and colonic irrigation in a clinic
- Herbal remedies
- Change your eating habits
- Detox with appropriate juices
- There are "colon cleansers" you can buy online

A good colon cleanser of your choice, along with appropriate foods and juices, should remove the toxins that are built up in your colon.

Your physician will be able to provide any further information on this topic.

How to prepare best a week pre-procedure

Before you live with the gastric balloon, let's say two weeks or, at the bare minimum, a week before you go to surgery, the surgeon will more than probably advise you to start dieting.

If you are like me, you could be thinking, "Right, I'm going to starve myself for six months, so I'd better eat everything I like right now and then lose weight with the gastric balloon."

WRONG.

Unless you are unlike me and know you are confident that you can adapt to another eating behaviour right away, please read on.

Our body doesn't have a "brain" the way we qualify a brain in the sense it doesn't think by itself, but it has an excellent memory. We can think of it as a computer. A computer doesn't think, but stores information in its internal memory.

This means that if you train your body to eat a lot and then starve itself because you want to slim down, it will panic and store up to make up for starvation mode. When you start eating again, it gets worse.

So, train your body to eat small portions regularly so that it doesn't panic and breaks down food whenever it's supposed to. Besides, by avoiding cravings, you will eat reasonably and not overindulge, especially in the evenings.

Eventually, remember that once the gastric balloon is inserted in your stomach, you won't feel that hungry, so balancing your day with small intakes of healthy foods before surgery is a good approach and won't shock your body in a few weeks.

Also, starting a diet will facilitate the placement of the balloon.

What to do the day prior to the procedure

Today is the day before surgery. You're going to be quite active today, in many ways. Remember that even though this surgery is not invasive, it is still an alien device that is going to be placed inside your stomach.

Your body is going to adjust to its new companion, but as in every adjustment, it takes a bit of time.

As a result, the first two to five, or even seven days, you often feel sick, dizzy, and tired.

Bearing this in mind, I did clean my place. You can do that, too, if you wish, knowing that you won't be able to do much during the coming week. I know, I thought the same, sorry to bring bad news! However, this is temporary. (I am not referring to the house cleaning here, only to the adjustment of the balloon.)

Now that this is done, you might want to shop for a few essentials like fruits, vegetables, milk, and mineral water to cover you for the next two days.

The first two days, you are not advised to eat anything solid or semi-solid, only liquids are recommended.

At this point, I bought a juice/soup/smoothie maker. You can, too, if you don't have one already.

The reason behind this is that preparing your own juices, smoothies, and soups can quickly become your daily routine. It has become mine.

You will have use for the liquid maker in the coming days as you are going to drink a lot of juices and after a short while, a lot of pureed fruits and smoothies.

Tonight, you are going to eat something light and you are going to ensure that you stop eating and drinking twelve hours before surgery.

How about having a juice mid-afternoon, a salad for dinner, plenty of water, and have an early night?

D-Day, what does the procedure entail?

Today is the big day. You might feel both excited and apprehensive. I know I was. There are so many questions popping into your head, right?

- Is the procedure going to hurt? Not at all, you will be sedated so you won't feel a thing. Also, your surgeon will sedate/numb your throat with a spray.

- How long is it going to take? On average it takes 20 to 30 minutes; mine took 25 minutes.

- How many people will there be in the theatre? Once the nurse has cleared, there is no contra-indication, and you have had a few tests done, you will be going to the theatre where you will be greeted by the surgeon, an anaesthetist, and a nurse. (Based on my own experience, this might vary according to the clinic's procedures.)

- How difficult is it to inflate the balloon? At the extremity of the balloon, there is a possibility to adjust a tube or catheter. This tube is going to help the surgeon insert the balloon, while it is still deflated, through the mouth and down the oesophagus until it reaches the stomach; this is called an endoscopy. Once inflated, the catheter is removed and the self-sealing valve will ensure the balloon is securely sealed and moves freely inside your stomach.

- What is the balloon filled with? It depends on the kind of gastric balloon you have opted for: it is either going to be filled with air or with a sterile saline solution.

- What is the capacity of the balloon's inflation? It depends on both your surgeon and yourself. You usually discuss this prior to the placement of the balloon as the inflation of the balloon has its importance to your weight loss. For instance, I had requested the balloon to be inflated to its maximum capacity to optimise my weight loss.

- How will I know if the balloon leaks? If you have opted for the liquid-filled balloon, the sterile saline solution is coloured. If you notice the colour of your urine turning green/blue, you must contact your physician to avoid any complications.

- What if I am worried or experiencing a strong pain? Remember that your physician is on call for twenty-four hours post procedure. However, this is very rare and after researching on different forums, I haven't read anything dramatic post procedure.

- Where am I going after the procedure? You will be moved into a recovery room until you wake up and the nurse can ensure all is okay. You will then be recovering in a semi-private or private room. Some hospitals/clinics request a few hours and then discharge you if you have no fever, etc. In other cases, the price includes a night's stay at the hospital as a standard practice. I stayed for a few hours and was discharged the same day.

- Am I seeing the surgeon again? Yes. He/she will validate the success of the procedure, tell you how long it took, check the tests the nurse will have performed post intervention (temperature, etc.)

before signing you off. The surgeon will also prescribe a course of oral medication, which will help in reducing the acidity in your stomach. I was given six months' worth of medication.

- <u>Can I drive after the procedure?</u> No. Either you get someone to accompany you, or you ensure you have a taxi to bring you home. I was very lucky to have a friend with me during that emotional adventure. She drove me to the clinic and stayed until she could drive me home. It was a great relief to know I could rely on someone.

- <u>What Shall I do when I get home?</u> Nothing! You will feel very sleepy, especially if you haven't spent an overnight stay at the hospital, so you will probably go straight to bed and rest.

- <u>Am I fit to go back to work in a few hours?</u> No. Some websites suggest you can resume work right after. This frustrates me, to be honest. None of my friends could resume work right after the balloon was fitted. In my opinion, it is unlikely that the people who write *we can resume work straight after* have had it implanted themselves. I was incapable of resuming work for a couple of days. That's why I ensured that I booked this procedure on a Friday so I had the whole weekend to rest and recuperate. I'm happy I did, because it is pure utopia to pretend you are fit for work a couple of hours after the procedure.

Chapter Nine

The First Day's Post Procedure

What are the possible symptoms?

Below is a list of all the symptoms you should be aware of and might encounter during the journey. They may occur during the first week, first three months, and/or last three months. All of them are natural and are to be expected, to some extent. You might not experience them all or, if you do, it might be very light symptoms or temporary symptoms. For the very first days, what are the symptoms?

- Nausea
- Vomiting
- Tiredness
- Dizziness
- Discomfort in the stomach
- Inability to eat

How to deal with them

- <u>Nausea and vomiting</u>: It is essential to keep hydrated, so drink or sip plenty of fluids like water and juices. I also drank lots of ginger tea. It also helped to apply a cold and humid towel on my forehead. Smelling mint and peppermint also helped.
- <u>Tiredness and dizziness</u>: Sleep, sleep, sleep. When you aren't sleeping, watch TV, lie down, and rest with no activity whatsoever.
- <u>Discomfort in the stomach</u>: This occurs especially when you try to get some sleep. Try not to lie down

completely. Instead, add a few pillows or elevate your bed and try to sleep on your left side or on your back. The point is for you to have your head higher than the level of the stomach.

- <u>Inability to eat</u>: As mentioned above, for the very first two days, you will be able to sip water, some juices, and perhaps eat some jelly. After two days, you will find yourself looking for something slightly more substantial such as smoothies, baby purees (well, that was my case), and yoghurt.

After a few days, I was eating small portions of brown rice with small bits of chicken breast, although hunger was almost inexistent.

Well done! You've done the most challenging part of your journey. It should only get easier now as time goes by.

Chapter Ten

What Are the Symptoms Within the First Three Months?

What are the possible symptoms/side effects?

During the first three months, you can experience some uneasy symptoms, which are more than likely to occur in the first few weeks. By this stage, the gastric balloon is becoming more familiar and in tune with your stomach and your body but is still in adaptation mode.

You could experience various degrees of the side effects mentioned below.

Let's have a look at the symptoms you may encounter during the first months of co-habitation:

- Nausea (rapidly fading away) / dizziness
- Tiredness / fatigue / lethargy
- Irritability
- Acid reflux (or more commonly called burps)
- Discomfort when sleeping (also fading with time)
- Abdominal bloating
- Diarrhoea
- Constipation

How to deal with them

You can apply the tips described in chapter nine for nausea. However, let's review the rest of the symptoms and what you can do to tackle them so that they do not affect you during your journey:

- Tiredness: Remember that you won't be able to keep your existing dietary habits and that your portions are going to be reduced considerably. The first days, or even weeks, you won't feel like doing much exercise. If you are normally very active, not exercising could increase tiredness. I took a course of vitamins and felt better after a while.

  When choosing, I opted for a vitamin a day containing all essential vitamins and nutrients. Vitamins I would recommend would be the ones containing magnesium, chromium, manganese, zinc, and vitamin B. A word on the tablets or pills: I struggled to swallow the tablets and had to resort to cutting them (with a pill cutter available at all leading pharmacies). This is the reason I have listed a multivitamin in liquid form.

- Irritability: You might not be irritable at all, but I was! I felt more vulnerable having to adjust to my new life without the help and encouragement of a support group. That would have been greatly beneficial. As a result, my feelings of isolation were more enhanced, because I had no one to turn to or share my experience with. Although many people I came into contact with were well intentioned, they couldn't relate to what I was going through. This led to my being irritable.

- Acid reflux: (or more commonly called burps): These, unfortunately, bring much discomfort and even embarrassment. The course of oral medication your surgeon will prescribe will help to an extent but will not totally dispel the burps. This was, for me, the most challenging symptom, so I made many attempts with food, etc. until I felt better. Ginger teas worked well for me. So did chewing my food a lot more. Reducing caffeine helped, too. Another tip that worked for me was eating rice (you can now find wholegrain Basmati rice) and eating beans. Avoid raw fruit straight after a meal. Instead, try cooking apples together with a pinch of cinnamon. Light exercises also helped.

- <u>Discomfort when sleeping</u>: (also fading away with time): Apart from elevating your head, you need to ensure you do not go to bed within two hours of eating. I have read many comments saying that the physician had recommended an eating time of 6 pm for dinner. I don't advocate that time as being the cut off time for dinner! As long as you adhere to the two hours period of time before going to bed, you should be fine. Fair enough in the UK or Ireland where people tend to have dinner early in the evening, but some cultures eat dinner around 8 pm, or even later, so eating at 6 pm would be too much of a change; and how about those who work late? You are on a weight management program, not in jail!

- <u>Abdominal Bloating</u>: You might feel bloated right after eating. Do not drink with your meal but outside your meals. It is equally important to drink before a meal and really important after a meal to clean the balloon. Think of it this way: drinking water a few minutes after a meal has the same effect as flushing toxins away. More on bloating later on when we review why a good understanding of digestion is important when you live with the stomach balloon.

- <u>Diarrhoea</u>: If you suffer from diarrhoea, the same regime applies as if you had no gastric balloon: bananas, rice, toast, and low-fibre foods are all good essential foods to include in your diet. Fruits, vegetables, and high-fibre foods are to be avoided.

- <u>Constipation</u>: Drink lots of water and homemade vegetable juices. Increase your fibre intake by opting for wholegrain bread, beans, and dried figs. You can also add prunes in yoghurt in the morning or as a snack. Remember, however, not to eat too much raw fruit on its own or straight after a meal, because although it will help to counteract constipation, it will trigger acid reflux.

Chapter Eleven

The Last Remaining Months with the Gastric Balloon

Possible symptoms/side effects and how to overcome them

You will notice that the side effects have switched from physical uncomfortable symptoms to your weight decreasing more slowly. This is because your balloon is now perfectly comfortable in your stomach and you co-habit perfectly well with it now.

Acid reflux could still be a nuisance though, but to a far lesser extent.

However, the whole point of having the gastric balloon inserted is to lose weight, right? So what's happened? How come weight loss seems to be decreasing after three months and reaches what is commonly known as a *plateau*?

First, you need to remember that your digestive system is even more important at this stage than in regular times.

This is because your stomach works harder with the device. This is the reason why you experienced a few symptoms at the start of the journey, but also the reason why you have lost weight rapidly the first two or three months, depending on how much the balloon was originally inflated.

Now however, the balloon is happily living in your stomach and it has started to decrease in volume and works less hard.

Luckily, by now you have benefited from nutritional, support, and therapeutic sessions, so you are on the right path. This doesn't prevent the dreaded plateau to start showing its insidious face though—that is all normal.

Please read the section on the plateau and how to successfully overcome it.

Chapter Twelve

Your Last Day with the Gastric Balloon

The same advice applied when you had the gastric balloon placed six months ago: you need to fast for twelve hours before having the balloon removed.

The procedure will entail basically the same process: you get a pre visit with the nurse, you then go to the theatre and are sedated. The only difference is that you could feel some discomfort when the surgeon removes the balloon, but it is all normal, nothing to be apprehensive about. I am mentioning this to you because I would have preferred to have been advised. I wondered if it was the normal procedure or not. It was.

You will rest a little bit in the semi-private or private room and then you will be discharged shortly after.

This will be a very exciting day for you, close to euphoria!

Many congratulations on your achievement!

Chapter Thirteen

Keep Up Your Great Efforts and Make It a Lifelong Journey!

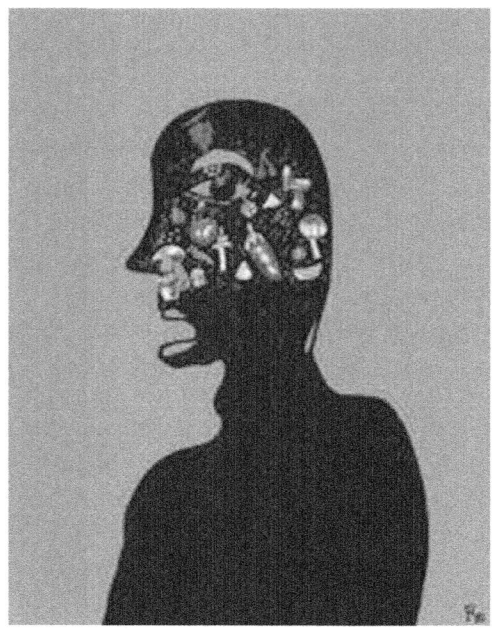

Make your healthy life a long-lasting routine

By now, you should have reached your realistic goal, which is an average of 20 kilos (slightly more than 3 stone or 44 pounds).

If you have achieved slightly less, that's okay too. The program doesn't stop with the removal of the gastric balloon:

- You now eat mainly low GI foods
- You drink plenty of water every day

- You chew your food properly
- You have reversed your resistance to insulin
- You have an exercise routine
- You also have a relaxation technique that works for you
- Thanks to the therapeutic sessions you have attended, you will not fall into the same trap again

Attend an additional therapy session if under pressure

At any time after the removal of the gastric balloon, if you feel that there is a danger you could be tempted by your old bad pattern, don't hesitate to have additional sessions with your therapist. <u>Don't let your body dictate your life; your mind is in control.</u>

Feel proud about the new YOU! You deserve it!

Chapter Fourteen

What Is the Plateau?

The dreaded plateau is simply the period during which you are not losing weight any more or the weight loss is slowing down. This period is more or less transitional, depending on how you manage it.

At this critical stage, some people are discouraged and feel there is nothing they can do that could help in overcoming the plateau. It is indeed tempting to believe that this is it: the maximum weight loss has been achieved, the plateau has kicked in, and we will stop losing weight. Instead, try to maintain the weight loss already achieved and kick-start the weight loss again!

There are solutions to counteract the plateau.

For now, I will just say that plateaus occur even though you are still following the diet and in some cases following some exercise routine. What worked before doesn't seem to be working any longer, hence the plateau.

Do we all hit the plateau?

I believe we all hit a plateau at some point. Some would hit that plateau when they have reached their desired BMI. This happens when you have only a few pounds to lose. For others, it happens during the course of the diet, knowing you still have some weight to lose and want to lose more weight.

Even celebrities follow the same path.

Actress Tina Malone, admitted in 2008, soon after having had the balloon implanted in March, that three months after the device was placed she had lost 3 stone and had reached a plateau. "The last month has been harder because the weight loss has slowed down."

Why do we hit the plateau with the gastric balloon program?

When you start the gastric diet, weight falls off because you eat regular, smallish portions, ideally levelling insulin out. In some cases, if you were not an advocate of drinking water and herbal teas, chances are that you have now increased your fluid intake. You might also have decided to take on some sort of exercise.

All this, ironically enough, even though you are doing all the right things, contributes to the creation of a plateau.

The fact that since day one you have been eating several small portions of food is, I believe, as I explain in this book, one of the positive effects of the balloon being placed in the stomach. Indeed, I do believe the ghrelin communicates quickly to the hypothalamus in our brain and indicates that satiety has been reached.

This is a quick reminder. The online *Medical News* explains:

> [...]"Ghrelin is a hormone produced mainly by [...] the human stomach and [...] stimulates hunger. Ghrelin levels increase before meals and decrease after meals. Ghrelin is also produced in the hypothalamic arcuate nucleous, where it stimulates the secretion of growth hormone from the anterior pituitary gland. [...]. Ghrelin plays a significant role in [...] the hippocampus, and is essential for

cognitive adaptation to changing environments and the process of learning.].

Considering the first months with the gastric balloon, I do think that by sharing the same space as the stomach, the balloon positively contributes to alerting the brain we had reached satiety pretty quickly. It is logical to think that after a few months, what was probably automatic due to a restricted space, is not automatic any longer and needs to be monitored and controlled.

In other words, I believe that having small portions could be challenging at this stage, during the plateau, unless your stomach has registered the small portions as being part of its routine and you don't feel the need to eat more.

This happened to me, although I started to crave some comfort foods. But, I didn't want to eat bigger portions of food. My stomach had gone into a comfortable routine of being satisfied with three small portions of food and two snacks.

In any case, I do believe that at this stage, we need to tame the ghrelin hormone.

Now, I would like to emphasise clearly the following, which is, I think, very interesting: different articles conclude that the ghrelin hormone is also triggered more significantly when the individual is under stress. The ghrelin hormone would then entice the individual to opt for comfort food.

This has been corroborated by the Mind Lab International Study when on 4 January 2010, in a Channel 4 TV show called *My Big Fat Diet*, the study revealed that responses in the brain dictated our behaviour to choose between healthy or comfort food. Comfort food is said to release a very high level of relaxation.

What does this mean to me?

To me, it means that we now know that the ghrelin hormone:

- Alerts the brain when we are hungry
- Releases higher levels under stress, which in turn leads to desiring comfort food

So for me, the plateau can be effectively counteracted by an efficient control of the ghrelin hormone: keep the food intake at regular times, including two snacks, in order to avoid any hunger pangs; try to reduce the amount of stress, which would otherwise lead to the consumption of comfort foods.

How to counteract the plateau

One of the successful ways of getting a new boost is by regulating the ghrelin hormone through the regular intake of appropriate foods in several smallish portions a day, including healthy snacks, and by keeping the ghrelin hormone happy with stress relief management techniques.

I have insisted on this concept because it is very important to grasp its principals in order to lead a successful, healthy life. So let's see.

A. Regulation of the ghrelin hormone with appropriate foods

Is there such a thing as *ghrelin foods*? YES and we are familiar with those foods. We've heard about them, read about them, and we can list a few foods off the top of our heads: low GI foods.

Low GI foods have a positive effect on our mood because they generate the neurotransmitter serotonin, which is the neurotransmitter acting on pain, appetite, mood, and sleep. You will find a few recipes in my *Gastric Diet* book.

B. Incorporate foods & drinks that boost your metabolism

Our metabolism is, in simple terms, the way our body ingests food and transforms it into energy. In other words, the more energy we burn, the more calories we burn. Weight loss is the direct result of boosting metabolism through some foods and drinks, and, as we will see later in this book, thanks to specific sportive movements.

Foods that contribute to boosting our metabolism are oats (does the Dukan diet ring a bell? Oats is one main aspect of his diet); whole grains; sardines, tuna, salmon, chicken, turkey (proteins—some diets immediately pop into mind); celery, cucumber, spinach; cinnamon; yoghurt; almonds; ginger; etc.

Drinks include (you will have guessed) water and green tea.

C. Keep the ghrelin hormone happy with stress relief management techniques

I will give you a few ideas, although you may already be on a routine.

Meditation: I like to meditate, and I have also included specific colours and aromatherapy during meditations.

For instance, I was offered an aroma diffuser, and I love it! It emits relaxing music (I particularly like listening to the sound of birds or ocean waves), diffuses the aromatherapy I pour at the start of a session, and displays a ray of colours throughout the hour. It directly connects to a few of my senses and the experience is just fantastic.

Yoga: I personally don't do yoga, but a few friends of mine swear by it and Pilates. They find both techniques a great way to relax while providing a good work out.

Reiki: I am a reiki master and have been practicing for a number of years. I am now practising on myself and feel really good after a session. I have included the weight loss factor in my sessions.

Listening to music: I dance quite a bit. When I don't, I listen to my MP3. I close my eyes and I feel great. My imagination wanders, and I fill my thoughts with happy ones and visualize myself with a great body!

These are only a few examples. Oh, and yes, sex as well.

Specific foods and stress reducing techniques all contribute to taming the ghrelin hormone.

D. Cortisol or the necessity to reduce stress levels

I know that when I was mentioning to my family and friends that reducing stress would be beneficial to weight loss, there were a few grins.

Of course, it is more widely accepted that reducing certain foods, increasing your intake of water and herbal teas and including some sort of regular exercise, however light the exercise might be, contribute to weight loss.

We have read it again and again. It's been demonstrated and medically proven.

So what's the deal about stress? Well, we have just explained the importance of taming the ghrelin hormone by also reducing the level of stress. Now, let's talk about cortisol. Suffice it to say that cortisol is typically referred to as the stress hormone that has many actions, such as blood pressure.

Its dysfunction can lead to weight gain (around the abdomen).

Are you with me? It would mean that reducing stress could consequently promote or have a positive effect on weight loss, at least in the abdominal area.

At this point, I need to ... *stress* ... that optimum digestion is critical if you want the balloon to happily cohabit in the stomach. Stress could also lead to excessive stomach acidity and, trust me, you certainly don't want this.

E. **Perform cardio and resistance interval training**

Last, but not least is cardio exercise, or better said, an ideal combination of cardio exercise alternated with resistance exercise and resting times.

When I first started the gastric diet, I was tired and in no condition to exercise much. I was walking and, after a while, I joined a few dance classes. But cardio exercise was not for me.

I was really motivated to lose weight, so I joined a gym for a little while. Because I had hit the plateau, I was working on a routine that my coach had developed for me. It was a total of 45 minutes broken down into an intense workout on the treadmill, a less intense workout on the treadmill, and another intense work out. I was then alternating with 10 minutes to build my back and leg muscles. Okay, not my favourite time, if I'm being honest, but the results were phenomenal. Note that it took approximately three weeks to start seeing a significant change in my body appearance.

Do you remember when we talked about metabolism? Well, boosting metabolism with foods is a must. The other way to speed up the weight loss and leave the plateau behind is by increasing your muscle mass. The more muscles you build, the more calories you burn—as muscles, even at rest, work hard and use a lot of calories.

At this stage, I should provide a word of caution: you might see that the scale doesn't change much, regardless of all the exercise you are doing. This doesn't mean you are not losing weight. It only means that you are building some muscles, getting rid of fat, and going in the right direction. After a few days, the weight should fall off again.

Chapter Fifteen

Some Physical Exercise

A word on sport

After two or three days, you will feel better. Everybody is different. Some friends felt better after one day while it took me about a week, on and off. Do not exercise; your body is still trying to adjust to its new life.

After two weeks, let's say, you can go for a walk and have a bit of fresh air, but again, remember that you are not supposed to train for the marathon! Be gentle with your body, with yourself. If you feel you can't walk more than five minutes, that's fine. That is still great.

Indeed, a small amount of regular exercise is the other step to a better lifestyle. After a while, you will feel like extending the walk to another five minutes and again five minutes.

I would urge you not to run or to practice any heavy sport. Remember, at that stage, you should have a BMI of around 30, and this means that you need to be gentle with your joints.

Before looking into what sportive activities you can join, a word on the gear, if I may, as it has greatly helped me:

- For us ladies, a good sports bra (sadly I had to change size due to the weight loss, but still, a wise buy).
- A good pair of tennis shoes (if you walk, why not try the MBT trainers! I love them. They tone you as you walk and you feel the difference. I feel I have

exercised twice as much, even though I have walked the same distance, when I wear MBT trainers or sketchers).

- Appropriate socks. I have sensitive feet in the sense that if I walk a lot, they get irritated and are prone to blistering, etc., so investing in pure cotton workout socks that are also heel cushioned will make a positive difference. I even found some toe socks! A little secret: for us women, a good pair of socks relates to a marathon in itself. Do you know where I usually buy my socks now? In the gents corner!!! How about that!

Now is the time to decide what kind of sport you want to practice, if you are not in a routine already.

This is quite exciting; there are many activities out there! Okay, in my case, I admit with shame that I am not a fan of dangerous things at all. Even the thought of skiing absolutely terrifies me, so does height. In fact, I'm not a fan of any sports, so I guess that this considerably restricted my enthusiasm to run out of the door and look for some excitement. But I did it. I did it because losing weight was all that mattered, and I am a very determined person.

I tried to read as much as I could in order to find out exactly what kind of gentle exercise I could practice in order to burn as many calories as I could and maximise my efforts in that respect.

Let's see: jogging burns up to 545 calories an hour.

Interesting.

Too bad I hate jogging.

Martial arts burn up to at least 280 calories an hour; perfect; no, wait: black eye and possibly a broken arm. I still need to look my best so maybe I need to avoid looking like I am just out of jail.

Okay, next. Swimming, now we're talking. Love water, love the fish; in this particular case, I swim without the fish, but still enjoy it and miracle, I also burn up to 300 calories an hour. I love my life. I became (not addicted, I won't fool anyone here) interested in aqua aerobics: you exercise for 45 minutes in the swimming pool, following the instructions of a person who shows you movements outside the pool. The beauty of that sport is that when your body is in water, you can't feel you are working out and there is no muscle pain.

Dancing is also part of my routine. I've been dancing since the age of eight years old. I love dancing. I love salsa and have discovered pretty recently another great Latin type of musical workout: Zumba. Maybe not the selection I would make to start with if you are not familiar with this kind of workout, but because I am used to dancing, I loved that option and now swear by it.

Actually, whether or not you want to shift the weight, it's a lot of fun! And it keeps your body in great shape once you have stabilised the ideal weight.

Another exciting exercise is walking as you can still burn up to 280 calories an hour— brisk walking that is. You can walk with a friend or, like me, take your MP3 and walk. I'm finding it surprisingly relaxing and refreshing at the same time. I bought a pedometer to keep me going. I got a basic one, but shop around as according to your budget, you can get one that not only calculates the number of steps, but also calculates the distance you have walked as well as the calories you have spent.

Of course, I was not walking every day and no, I can see what you're thinking, that I was lazy. That is not the reason. The reason is that when you live in England, you can tick on your calendar the days it's not raining. You need to understand: make-up, hair, nice training jumpsuit ... and after all the effort, I absolutely cannot look like I have come out of the gutter with my make-up running awkwardly along my face, with my hair sticking as if I hadn't washed it for a week. After all, one needs to keep some standards.

Ah yes, the gym. I see your point.

This is an achievement for me, because let me tell you that exercising was not part of my life before the gastric balloon. When friends were asking me if I wanted to take part in any kind of physical, foreseeable muscular pain activity, I was simply replying that I would take the car and meet them at their destination, or one of my favourite quotes was "I don't walk, I don't run, I glide, thank you very much." Well, now I walk. I will never run, but I do walk.

Chapter Sixteen

Travelling Tips

Tips if you travel

First of all, my concern was to know if I could travel with the gastric balloon fitted in my stomach, especially during the first three months.

The answer was: Yes. It is safe to travel with a fitted gastric balloon fitted in the stomach.

Actually, for the six months I had the balloon fitted in my stomach, I was travelling quite a fair bit with my work. After getting reassurance, I got on a flight shortly after the placement of the balloon. It was a short haul, and it was an upsetting tummy experience. So, here are some tips to avoid the same experience and ensure that yours is optimised.

I decided to write a section around flights because a friend of mine who was interested in getting the gastric balloon fitted, but whose job involved lots of travelling, was concerned about its safety and experience.

It's true that we tend to travel quite a bit for work or leisure, or both. However, despite the fact that airlines are always adding new destinations to their websites, correct me if I'm wrong, most airline companies haven't thought of offering alternative meals.

It's all about being cost effective.

I used to have a free meal or a sandwich of some kind on some airlines. Now, if I want to get something, I need to buy it. The same goes for drinks. I'm talking economy here because in first class, you still have your meal (although I will confess I don't know if for the same flight you still have foie gras for instance).

My point is that flying is pretty common nowadays, but I am still not offered a low calorie or healthy alternative for a meal. Usually, it's the choice between being vegetarian or not, when there's a choice at all.

Tips for short hauls

As I mentioned, on short hauls, I used to get sandwiches (still do with some airlines) and nearly fall off my seat every time by the suspicious look of them—because of the fat content and the cheap spongy kind of bread. Thank God my seat belt is always fastened!

If, when booking my flight, I was given the option to choose a healthy alternative, I would tick the box for sure, even if that meant a little extra from my pocket. That's another factor to take into consideration, the economic one, where healthy options or healthy foods are usually more expensive. Shame. Does this mean I have to go fishing myself, run after the chickens of my neighbours, and grow my own vegetables? Maybe I will.

Anyway, the first flight I took after having the gastric balloon placed, I just didn't think twice. All I wanted to ensure was my safety on the flight, not on the kind of food and drink I should consider.

On some flights, I'm offered very salty nibbles or sugary ones. On that flight I had the delightful choice of the chicken sandwich or the vegetarian sandwich. Because I'm not a vegetarian, I opted for the chicken one. Oh dear, I'm supposed to be smart, right? No brain on that flight for sure. Bottom line, I nearly passed out. I didn't know if I had just agreed to get a sandwich with butter or with anything else. I still remember to this day the excruciating moment when I bit the sandwich and immediately looked around to see if I was going to be seen as my hand nervously headed for the airsick bag to vomit the butter sandwich—never again.

So, what are the alternatives

A. Prepare a wrap or a bite at home and bring it with you to the airport. Don't pack any liquids, though, as they will be confiscated.

B. Try to eat at home or at the canteen at work if possible.

C. Check the menus that are usually displayed outside the restaurants at the airport. At some airports you have seafood and light meals. Light meals could include dips such as raita (yogurt with garlic and mint, sometimes with cucumber chunks) and babaganoush (aubergine puree) with raw vegetables; or some tapas such as gambas, potatoes, seafood, a small plate of paella, or pasta with aubergines and courgette in a tomato sauce. A seafood cocktail is good when the mayonnaise can be left on the side. Remember to allow some time to chew and optimise your digestion. Also, remember the principles detailed in the gastric balloon diet with the right combination of foods.

D. There are some natural and fresh juices and smoothies' booths at many airports that could be a good alternative, especially during the first month of the placement of the balloon, when your hunger is considerably reduced and yet you crave fresh fruits. When you get a smoothie or a juice, remember that you can ask to have ginger added, for instance.

E. Choose a healthy wrap and some water or fruit at the convenient stores located inside the airport. Some could offer crab or salmon on brown granary bread, wild rice salad with lentils and tomatoes, pasta salad with tomatoes, and peppers.

F. If you have unwanted symptoms, such as nausea, a mint could do the trick. Please stay away from chewing gums that could create gas. Another tip is to massage your hands.

G. Do you have a pass for a visit to the lounge? Good. But this is not a reason to be careless in your choice of food and drink. Lounges have a tendency to offer a lot of snacks and wine. Although very tempting, it is best to avoid those. You have the choice, however, as most of the time you can choose. It is sometimes an open plan: water, brown bread sandwiches, if any, and orange juice (not from concentrate). Lounges should be considered more for the experience than for food and drink. In there, you can relax; read newspapers and magazines; read notifications about flights; and the sofas and couches are very comfortable. It's a relaxing experience and I love them, but not the most memorable culinary experience, for me anyway.

H. On the flight itself, avoid the saggy sandwich which is usually full of butter and could make you feel nauseous and upset your stomach the same way it did to me. But, by all means, take water, tomato juice, water with a slice of lemon, or something you enjoy.

You need to include some pleasurable moments, otherwise it will be quite tough to observe a very strict diet at all times! Personally, after a few weeks, I was allowing myself a small bottle of red wine, but I could only drink half the bottle. It is even better if you fly with a colleague, a friend, a family member, or your better half. You could ask for a second glass and take a sip or two, enough to please your palate without compromising on your diet. (The same goes in restaurants, at home, etc.)

Tips for long hauls

You are in luck if you travel long hauls. I am usually offered—in advance—a choice of meals and because there is variety there, I can always discard a few ingredients and eat the rest. So long hauls are great, to me anyway. I have flown with probably ten airlines and have always enjoyed some options.

Conclusion

I hope you have enjoyed this book and feel ready to embark on such an exciting and life-changing adventure!

You have made the right decision. If I had to do it all over again, I would do it, only sooner.

After I finished this first book, I was asked if I could help further by sharing all the recipes I had developed during this adventure. I wrote it and am sharing with you recipes that have worked for me. I have also made sure they are all packed with great taste! It's called "*My Successful Gastric Balloon Diet – 4 Steps to Lose Weight and Keep it Off*!"

Not only this, but I was also asked what was allowed to eat when socialising and entertaining, if take outs were a no-no; so I have written a book on this and it's nearly ready! I will publish it in January, but you can prebook it here: "*My Top-secret Socialising Tips with the Gastric Balloon – Entertain, eat out, and enjoy take-outs*!"

Christmas is a fabulous time, but it can be daunting if you don't know what to eat and drink with the gastric balloon. Fear no more! "*How to Lose Weight Over Christmas with the Gastric Balloon – My tested, easy, and effective recipes*!" is being published in December, so that you can enjoy this festive season to the fullest!

I am currently working on another mini book around recipes for busy professionals. Stay tuned!

Is there a specific subject with regard to the gastric balloon you are interested in, or concerns you would like to share? I will be happy to hear from you at: supportgballoon@outlook.com

I wish you success and happiness with the new YOU!!

About the Author

Books by Sabine Fontaine:

How I lost Weight with the Gastric Balloon Program – Secrets and tips to a successful journey!

My Successful Gastric Balloon Diet – 4 steps to lose weight and keep it off!

How to Lose Weight at Christmas with the Gastric Balloon.

These books were conceived during her experience with the gastric balloon and were published over five years later to assess if it was a successful long-term weight-loss method.

The reason she is emphasising that this is a journey and not a standalone product is intentional as she finds it is critical to attend a support group and follow a therapy.

Sabine has a passion for on-going studies and learning in general—she holds a Master's Degree in Spanish with honours and a Master's Degree in International Trade with honours. Additionally, Sabine certified as a Reiki & Seichem Master, as an Indian Head Massage Therapist, and more recently as a Nutritionist. Finally, she certified in Hypnotherapy and in NLP (Neuro-Linguistic Programming) to try to understand how the mind works.

Sabine's ultimate goal is to provide effective help with weight loss and clearly explain how the combination of the gastric balloon together with a support group and behavioural changes leads to a long-term, perfect weight.

She welcomes your comments and thoughts about this book. Please email them to: supportgballoon@outlook.com

Printed in Great Britain
by Amazon